CODY SMITH

8 Weeks to 150 Consecutive Dips

Build up Your Upper Body Working Your Chest, Shoulders, and Triceps

First edition

ISBN: 978-1-952381-14-0

This book was professionally typeset on Reedsy.
Find out more at reedsy.com

Contents

Before You Begin

Hey reader, thanks for grabbing a copy of the book.

If you are looking to pair this workout program with a complimentary guide to shed weight and boost your growth hormones to build more muscle faster, then I have got you covered.

Seems crazy to do both at the same time, but you can.

Better still, it is stupid easy.

Oh, and it is free. You can do this method anytime you want, anywhere for the rest of your life.

I usually sell this information, but I want you to have it.

You can get a copy from your cell phone from a simple text.

Seriously, get your phone out and text BOOST to (678) 506-7543.

Cheers!

Introduction - How to Use This Book

Your body is truly the only gym you need to either tone up or build muscle.

People far too often think they need special equipment or heavy weights to see results.

Of course, who can blame them? Every gym and late-night infomercial have convinced us that to see results, we need something else that we do not have now to make it happen.

Luckily, if you have a body, you have a gym. And if you have a gym, you have access to results.

Just as long as you put in the work.

This program, like most of my programs, focuses on one exercise to target multiple muscles groups to see results.

Dips certainly fit that category and the next 8 weeks are going to be a gnarly ride to get to the finish line to complete 150 consecutive dips.

We are going to develop your chest, triceps, upper back, and, most importantly, your shoulders.

You see, shoulders are the gateway muscle. Everything upper body motion must pass through the shoulders to make it happen. You could have the biggest triceps and chest around but if your shoulders are weak...sorry boss, your shoulders are holding you back from your full potential.

What people do not realize is dips can be your "secret sauce" to upping your gains and staying out of plateaus across the board.

And sadly, you would be hard pressed to find a lot of people even in a gym who can do even 30 consecutive dips.

But we are not here to shoot for a mere 30. We are going straight for 150. A feat hardly anyone can do.

And that is exactly what we are going to tackle here in this 8-week program.

Sure, you could do dips on your own, try and knock out as many as possible every day and work your way to 150 but you are either going to fall short or give up before you even get there.

What you need is strategically designed workouts for your current fitness level that challenge you just enough without killing you. Each workout will push you for the proper progression to make steady gains along the way. This program is structured to take all the guesswork out of your journey to 150 consecutive dips.

You will just need access to some parallel bars to complete your dips. Just promise me you will not use some janky makeshift dip bars.

You will begin your journey with an initial assessment to determine your current max dip count. From there, you will be guided to your first workout to get started.

Once you complete the program, you will have earned the right to attempt the 150 dips in a row. Some people knock it out in the first attempt. Others need a few more weeks of training.

Now, I will warn you, these workouts can feel very repetitive at times. Far too often people look for variety and complexity to see results when really the simplest approach is best.

100 dips variations and off the wall workout routines are not what is going to get you to the results you want.

Showing up and putting in the work; that is where the real bacon is.

Some of you will not need the entire 8 weeks. Others will need more than 8 weeks. Either way is perfectly fine and doesn't mean the program doesn't work, it just means everyone comes from a different level of fitness.

8 weeks is not some magical number that will work for every single person. 8 weeks is the average amount of time it will take the average person to reach 150 consecutive dips so do not get too caught up in the timeline. It will take you however long that it takes you.

What I can promise you is if you put in the work, you will see the results.

Up next is the initial assessment. Get after it, champ.

Initial Dip Assessment

This is the first step into your incredible journey to doing 150 consecutive dips. It will be hard but manageable as you embark on something that very few people on the face of the earth have ever accomplished.

We are going to start out with a dip assessment to determine where you should start in the program.

As you can imagine, you will need dip bars to complete your assessment so go ahead and find some handy to get started.

Make sure you are doing full dips going all the way through the motion. Proper form is key to getting the most out of this exercise so I'll quickly go over how to properly perform a dip.

To perform a dip, grab the parallel dip bars and jump up into a straight arm hold. Descend your body by bending your arms as your lean forward. Gradually descend until your shoulders are just below your elbows. Ascend back up to the starting position with your arms straight but not locked. That is one rep.

Go ahead and complete as many correct dips as you can without stopping.

Once you are done, remember the number of fully completed dips and head to the post assessment results section.

Note: If this is the first assessment, you will write your assessment number in the '1st assessment' row. When you come back to do another assessment, you write in your completed number of reps in the respective row depending on how many assessments you have completed.

_____ reps: 1st assessment

_____ reps: 2nd assessment

_____ reps: 3rd assessment

_____ reps: 4th assessment

_____ reps: 5th assessment

_____ reps: 6th assessment

_____ reps: 7th assessment

_____ reps: 8th assessment

_____ reps: 9th assessment

_____ reps: 10th assessment

_____ reps: 11th assessment

_____ reps: 12th assessment

_____ reps: 13th assessment

_____ reps: 14th assessment

_____ reps: 15th assessment

_____ reps: 16th assessment

_____ reps: 17th assessment

_____ reps: 18th assessment

_____ reps: 19th assessment

_____ reps: 20th assessment

Post-Assessment Results

So... how did you do?

Were you surprised with how many you did or were you underwhelmed and disappointed that you did not do so hot?

Do not beat yourself up. This is simply a baseline for you to start from.

Go ahead and jog your memory of your assessment score.

With that score in mind, you are now going to be directed to your workout Grouping based on your score.

Do not get too caught up in the name of each group of workouts, these are just fun names to identify which group you are currently in. If you do not like your current group name, do not worry, stick with the program long enough and you will be out of that group in no time and into another group whose name you probably will not like either.

Before I go into informing you of your baseline workout, I recommend leaving a day between now and hitting your first workout to recover from your assessment. However, you do not have to if you are feeling gung-ho and want to go ahead and knock out your first workout.

- If you did less than 8, you will start in the foundations group to build up your strength.
- If you did 8, you will start in the Novice Group.
- If you did between 9 and 15, you will start in the Newb Group.
- If you did between 16 and 23, you will start in the Greenhorn Group.
- If you did between 24 and 30, you will start in the Cub Group.
- If you did between 31 and 38, you will start in the Rookie Group.
- If you did between 39 and 45, you will start in the Pleb Group.
- If you did between 46 and 53, you will start in the Gorilla Group.
- If you did between 54 and 60, you will start in the Viking Group.
- If you did between 61 and 68, you will start in the Elite Group.
- If you did between 69 and 75, you will start in the Commando Group.
- If you did between 76 and 84, you will start in the Veteran Group.
- If you did greater than 84, you will start in the Nuclear Group.

Now that you know your group, you know where you will begin for your next workout.

In your group, you will start with workout 1 followed by workout 2 and 3.

For example, let's say you completed 23 reps and you were going to workout Monday, Wednesday and Friday. That would put you in the Greenhorn Group with workout 1 on Monday, Workout 2 on Wednesday, and workout 3 on Friday.

The following week, you would start with Greenhorn Group Workout 4 followed by 5 and 6.

Simple enough.

Also, some of your workouts will involve what I call fundamental dips.

Fundamental dips involve a very slow descend and a normal ascend during the dip exercise. These work the full range of muscles throughout the entire dips. Typical dips only provide significant tensions when you raise your body from the floor. These dips make you work during the descent and the rise. You will have either 5 or 10 second descends during your workouts.

For example, if you have a set of 3 fundamental dips with 5 seconds descends, you will start in the up, ready position and lower yourself slowly over a 5 second period to the bottom of the exercise. You will then push back up to the starting position like a normal dip. As soon as you get to the top of the exercise, you will begin gradually lowering yourself back down over another 5 second period for the second rep followed by the third.

They do not sound bad, but boy do they start to burn quick.

Great job on your assessment and get ready for your first workout.

Workout Completion Checklist

Check off your workouts as you complete them:

_____Foundation Group Workout 1

_____Foundation Group Workout 2

_____Foundation Group Workout 3

_____Foundation Group Workout 4

_____Foundation Group Workout 5

_____Foundation Group Workout 6

_____Novice Group Workout 1

_____Novice Group Workout 2

_____Novice Group Workout 3

_____Novice Group Workout 4

_____Novice Group Workout 5

_____Novice Group Workout 6

_____Newb Group Workout 1

_____Newb Group Workout 2

_____Newb Group Workout 3

_____Newb Group Workout 4

_____Newb Group Workout 5

_____Newb Group Workout 6

_____Greenhorn Group Workout 1

_____Greenhorn Group Workout 2

_____Greenhorn Group Workout 3

_____Greenhorn Group Workout 4

_____Greenhorn Group Workout 5

_____Greenhorn Group Workout 6

_____Cub Group Workout 1

_____Cub Group Workout 2

_____Cub Group Workout 3

_____Cub Group Workout 4

_____Cub Group Workout 5

_____Cub Group Workout 6

_____Rookie Group Workout 1

_____Rookie Group Workout 2

_____Rookie Group Workout 3

_____Rookie Group Workout 4

_____Rookie Group Workout 5

_____Rookie Group Workout 6

_____Pleb Group Workout 1

_____Pleb Group Workout 2

_____Pleb Group Workout 3

_____Pleb Group Workout 4

_____Pleb Group Workout 5

_____Pleb Group Workout 6

_____Gorilla Group Workout 1

_____Gorilla Group Workout 2

_____Gorilla Group Workout 3

_____Gorilla Group Workout 4

_____Gorilla Group Workout 5

_____Gorilla Group Workout 6

_____Viking Group Workout 1

_____Viking Group Workout 2

_____Viking Group Workout 3

_____Viking Group Workout 4

_____Viking Group Workout 5

_____Viking Group Workout 6

_____Elite Group Workout 1

_____Elite Group Workout 2

_____Elite Group Workout 3

_____Elite Group Workout 4

_____Elite Group Workout 5

_____Elite Group Workout 6

_____Commando Group Workout 1

_____Commando Group Workout 2

_____Commando Group Workout 3

_____Commando Group Workout 4

_____Commando Group Workout 5

_____Commando Group Workout 6

_____Veteran Group Workout 1

_____Veteran Group Workout 2

_____Veteran Group Workout 3

_____Veteran Group Workout 4

_____Veteran Group Workout 5

_____Veteran Group Workout 6

_____Nuclear Group Workout 1

_____Nuclear Group Workout 2

_____Nuclear Group Workout 3

_____Nuclear Group Workout 4

_____Nuclear Group Workout 5

_____Nuclear Group Workout 6

_____Attempting 150 Consecutive Dips

_____Completed 150 Consecutive Dips: _____ reps.

Pre & Post Program Measurements

The following measurements are 100% optional and are not required to start or finish the program. I know some people will be curious to know other areas that are positively affected by achieving 150 consecutive dips.

Starting weight: _____

Starting dip rep max: _____

Starting push-up rep max: _____

Starting shoulder press max: _____

Starting bench press max: _____

Ending weight: _____

Ending dip rep max: _____

Ending push-up rep max: _____

Ending shoulder press max: _____

Ending bench press max: _____

Foundation Group Workouts

Foundation Group Workout 1

Welcome to the Foundation Group Workout 1.

For this workout, we have 5 sets with 60 seconds of rest between each set consisting of negative dips.

Negative dips simply focus on a slow descent without ascending to the up position. This means as soon as you complete your descent, you can stop and rest.

Remember to focus on proper form throughout your sets and always start on the up, ready position.

Sets:

1. 1 negative dip with a 3 second descend.
2. 1 negative dip with a 3 second descend.
3. 1 negative dip with a 3 second descend.
4. 1 negative dip with a 3 second descend.
5. 1 negative dip with a 3 second descend.

If you completed this workout, head to Foundation Group Workout 2 for your next session. If not, stick with this one until you complete it.

Foundation Group Workout 2

Welcome to the Foundation Group Workout 2.

For this workout, we have 5 sets with 60 seconds of rest between each set consisting of negative dips.

Remember to focus on proper form throughout your sets and always start in the up, ready position.

Sets:

1. 1 negative dip with a 3 second descend.
2. 1 negative dip with a 5 second descend.
3. 1 negative dip with a 5 second descend.
4. 1 negative dip with a 3 second descend.
5. 1 negative dip with a 3 second descend.

If you completed this workout, head to Foundation Group Workout 3 for your next session. If not, stick with this one until you complete it.

Foundation Group Workout 3

Welcome to the Foundation Group Workout 3.

For this workout, we have 5 sets with 60 seconds of rest between each set consisting of negative dips.

Remember to focus on proper form throughout your sets and always start in the up, ready position.

Sets:

1. 1 negative dip with a 5 second descend.
2. 1 negative dip with a 5 second descend.
3. 1 negative dip with a 5 second descend.
4. 1 negative dip with a 5 second descend.
5. 1 negative dip with a 5 second descend.

If you completed this workout, head to Foundation Group Workout 4 for your next session. If not, stick with this one until you complete it.

Foundation Group Workout 4

Welcome to the Foundation Group Workout 4.

For this workout, we have 5 sets with 60 seconds of rest between each set consisting of negative dips.

Remember to focus on proper form throughout your sets and always start in the up, ready position.

Sets:

1. 1 negative dip with a 5 second descend.
2. 1 negative dip with a 5 second descend.
3. 1 negative dip with a 7 second descend.
4. 1 negative dip with a 7 second descend.
5. 1 negative dip with a 7 second descend.

If you completed this workout, head to Foundation Group Workout 5 for your next session. If not, stick with this one until you complete it.

Foundation Group Workout 5

Welcome to the Foundation Group Workout 5.

For this workout, we have 5 sets with 60 seconds of rest between each set consisting of negative dips.

Remember to focus on proper form throughout your sets and always start in the up, ready position.

Sets:

1. 1 negative dip with a 7 second descend.
2. 1 negative dip with a 7 second descend.
3. 1 negative dip with a 7 second descend.
4. 1 negative dip with a 7 second descend.
5. 1 negative dip with a 7 second descend.

If you completed this workout, head to Foundation Group Workout 6 for your next session. If not, stick with this one until you complete it.

Foundation Group Workout 6

Welcome to the Foundation Group Workout 6.

For this workout, we have 5 sets with 60 seconds of rest between each set consisting of negative dips.

Remember to focus on proper form throughout your sets and always start in the up, ready position.

Sets:

1. 1 negative dip with a 10 second descend.
2. 1 negative dip with a 10 second descend.
3. 1 negative dip with a 10 second descend.
4. 1 negative dip with a 10 second descend.
5. 1 negative dip with a 10 second descend.

Since this is the end of a two-week period, it is time to redo your dip assessment to check your progress. Rest a day and give the assessment a go to see which Group you will be in next.

Novice Group Workouts

Novice Group Workout 1

Welcome to the Novice Group Workout 1.

For this workout, you have 6 sets with 60 seconds of rest between each set.

Remember to focus on proper form throughout your sets.

Sets:

1. 3 dips
2. 3 dips
3. 3 dips
4. 3 dips
5. 3 dips
6. 1 fundamental dip with a 5 second descend.

If you completed this workout, head to Novice Group Workout 2 for your next session. If not, stick with this one until you complete it.

Glasses of water drank today: 1-2-3-4-5-6-7-8-9-10

Hours of sleep last night: 1-2-3-4-5-6-7-8-9-10

Diet: junk food————semi-healthy————healthy

Novice Group Workout 2

Welcome to the Novice Group Workout 2.

For this workout, we have 6 sets with 60 seconds of rest between each set.

Remember to focus on proper form throughout your sets.

Sets:

1. 5 dips
2. 5 dips
3. 5 dips
4. 5 dips
5. 5 dips
6. 1 fundamental dip with a 5 second descend.

If you completed this workout, head to Novice Group Workout 3 for your next session. If not, stick with this one until you complete it.

Glasses of water drank today: 1-2-3-4-5-6-7-8-9-10

Hours of sleep last night: 1-2-3-4-5-6-7-8-9-10

Diet: junk food—————semi-healthy—————healthy

Novice Group Workout 3

Welcome to the Novice Group Workout 3.

For this workout, we have 6 sets with 90 seconds of rest between each set.

Remember to focus on proper form throughout your sets.

Sets:

1. 6 dips
2. 6 dips
3. 6 dips
4. 6 dips
5. 6 dips
6. Max out: perform as many dips as you can.

Max reps: _____

If you completed this workout, head to Novice Group Workout 4 for your next session. If not, stick with this one until you complete it.

Glasses of water drank today: 1-2-3-4-5-6-7-8-9-10

Hours of sleep last night: 1-2-3-4-5-6-7-8-9-10

Diet: junk food—————semi-healthy—————healthy

Novice Group Workout 4

Welcome to the Novice Group Workout 4.

For this workout, we have 6 sets with 60 seconds of rest between each set.

Remember to focus on proper form throughout your sets.

Sets:

1. 7 dips
2. 7 dips
3. 7 dips
4. 7 dips
5. 7 dips
6. 1 fundamental dip with a 5 second descend.

If you completed this workout, head to Novice Group Workout 5 for your next session. If not, stick with this one until you complete it.

Glasses of water drank today: 1-2-3-4-5-6-7-8-9-10

Hours of sleep last night: 1-2-3-4-5-6-7-8-9-10

Diet: junk food————semi-healthy————healthy

Novice Group Workout 5

Welcome to the Novice Group Workout 5.

For this workout, we have 6 sets with 60 seconds of rest between each set.

Remember to focus on proper form throughout your sets.

Sets:

1. 8 dips
2. 8 dips
3. 8 dips
4. 8 dips
5. 8 dips
6. 1 fundamental dip with a 5 second descend.

If you completed this workout, head to Novice Group Workout 6 for your next session. If not, stick with this one until you complete it.

Glasses of water drank today: 1-2-3-4-5-6-7-8-9-10

Hours of sleep last night: 1-2-3-4-5-6-7-8-9-10

Diet: junk food————semi-healthy————healthy

Novice Group Workout 6

Welcome to the Novice Group Workout 6.

For this workout, we have 6 sets with 90 seconds of rest between each set.

Remember to focus on proper form throughout your sets.

Sets:

1. 10 dips
2. 10 dips
3. 10 dips
4. 10 dips
5. 10 dips
6. Max out: perform as many dips as you can.

Max reps: _____

Since this is the end of a two-week period, it is time to redo your dip assessment to check your progress if you fully completed this workout.

Rest a day and give the assessment a go to see which Group you will be in next.

Glasses of water drank today: 1-2-3-4-5-6-7-8-9-10

Hours of sleep last night: 1-2-3-4-5-6-7-8-9-10

Diet: junk food———————semi-healthy———————healthy

Newb Group Workouts

Newb Group Workout 1

Welcome to the Newb Group Workout 1.

For this workout, we have 6 sets with 60 seconds of rest between each set.

Remember to focus on proper form throughout your sets.

Sets:

1. 8 dips
2. 8 dips
3. 8 dips
4. 8 dips
5. 8 dips
6. 1 fundamental dip with a 5 second descend.

If you completed this workout, head to Newb Group Workout 2 for your next session. If not, stick with this one until you complete it.

Glasses of water drank today: 1-2-3-4-5-6-7-8-9-10

Hours of sleep last night: 1-2-3-4-5-6-7-8-9-10

Diet: junk food————semi-healthy————healthy

Newb Group Workout 2

Welcome to the Newb Group Workout 2.

For this workout, we have 6 sets with 60 seconds of rest between each set.

Remember to focus on proper form throughout your sets.

Sets:

1. 10 dips
2. 10 dips
3. 10 dips
4. 10 dips
5. 10 dips
6. 1 fundamental dip with a 5 second descend.

If you completed this workout, head to Newb Group Workout 3 for your next session. If not, stick with this one until you complete it.

Glasses of water drank today: 1-2-3-4-5-6-7-8-9-10

Hours of sleep last night: 1-2-3-4-5-6-7-8-9-10

Diet: junk food————semi-healthy————healthy

Newb Group Workout 3

Welcome to the Newb Group Workout 3.

For this workout, we have 6 sets with 90 seconds of rest between each set.

Remember to focus on proper form throughout your sets.

Sets:

1. 12 dips
2. 12 dips
3. 12 dips
4. 12 dips
5. 12 dips
6. Max out: perform as many dips as you can.

Max reps: _____

If you completed this workout, head to Newb Group Workout 4 for your next session. If not, stick with this one until you complete it.

Glasses of water drank today: 1-2-3-4-5-6-7-8-9-10

Hours of sleep last night: 1-2-3-4-5-6-7-8-9-10

Diet: junk food————semi-healthy————healthy

Newb Group Workout 4

Welcome to the Newb Group Workout 4.

For this workout, we have 6 sets with 60 seconds of rest between each set.

Remember to focus on proper form throughout your sets.

Sets:

1. 14 dips
2. 14 dips
3. 14 dips
4. 14 dips
5. 14 dips
6. 1 fundamental dip with a 5 second descend.

If you completed this workout, head to Newb Group Workout 5 for your next session. If not, stick with this one until you complete it.

Glasses of water drank today: 1-2-3-4-5-6-7-8-9-10

Hours of sleep last night: 1-2-3-4-5-6-7-8-9-10

Diet: junk food————semi-healthy————healthy

Newb Group Workout 5

Welcome to the Newb Group Workout 5.

For this workout, we have 6 sets with 60 seconds of rest between each set.

Remember to focus on proper form throughout your sets.

Sets:

1. 15 dips
2. 15 dips
3. 15 dips
4. 15 dips
5. 15 dips
6. 2 fundamental dips with a 5 second descend.

If you completed this workout, head to Newb Group Workout 6 for your next session. If not, stick with this one until you complete it.

Glasses of water drank today: 1-2-3-4-5-6-7-8-9-10

Hours of sleep last night: 1-2-3-4-5-6-7-8-9-10

Diet: junk food—————semi-healthy—————healthy

Newb Group Workout 6

Welcome to the Newb Group Workout 6.

For this workout, we have 6 sets with 90 seconds of rest between each set.

Remember to focus on proper form throughout your sets.

Sets:

1. 17 dips
2. 17 dips
3. 17 dips
4. 17 dips
5. 17 dips
6. Max out: perform as many dips as you can.

Max reps: _____

Since this is the end of a two-week period, it is time to redo your dip assessment to check your progress if you fully completed this workout.

Rest a day and give the assessment a go to see which Group you will be in next.

Glasses of water drank today: 1-2-3-4-5-6-7-8-9-10

Hours of sleep last night: 1-2-3-4-5-6-7-8-9-10

Diet: junk food————semi-healthy————healthy

Greenhorn Group Workouts

Greenhorn Group Workout 1

Welcome to the Greenhorn Group Workout 1.

For this workout, we have 6 sets with 60 seconds of rest between each set.

Remember to focus on proper form throughout your sets.

Sets:

1. 14 dips
2. 14 dips
3. 14 dips
4. 14 dips
5. 14 dips
6. 1 fundamental dip with a 5 second descend.

If you completed this workout, head to Greenhorn Group Workout 2 for your next session. If not, stick with this one until you complete it.

Glasses of water drank today: 1-2-3-4-5-6-7-8-9-10

Hours of sleep last night: 1-2-3-4-5-6-7-8-9-10

Diet: junk food————semi-healthy————healthy

Greenhorn Group Workout 2

Welcome to the Greenhorn Group Workout 2.

For this workout, we have 6 sets with 60 seconds of rest between each set.

Remember to focus on proper form throughout your sets.

Sets:

1. 15 dips
2. 15 dips
3. 15 dips
4. 15 dips
5. 15 dips
6. 2 fundamental dips with a 5 second descend.

If you completed this workout, head to Greenhorn Group Workout 3 for your next session. If not, stick with this one until you complete it.

Glasses of water drank today: 1-2-3-4-5-6-7-8-9-10

Hours of sleep last night: 1-2-3-4-5-6-7-8-9-10

Diet: junk food—————semi-healthy—————healthy

Greenhorn Group Workout 3

Welcome to the Greenhorn Group Workout 3.

For this workout, we have 6 sets with 90 seconds of rest between each set.

Remember to focus on proper form throughout your sets.

Sets:

1. 17 dips
2. 17 dips
3. 17 dips
4. 17 dips
5. 17 dips
6. Max out: perform as many dips as you can.

Max reps: _____

If you completed this workout, head to Greenhorn Group Workout 4 for your next session. If not, stick with this one until you complete it.

Glasses of water drank today: 1-2-3-4-5-6-7-8-9-10

Hours of sleep last night: 1-2-3-4-5-6-7-8-9-10

Diet: junk food————semi-healthy————healthy

Greenhorn Group Workout 4

Welcome to the Greenhorn Group Workout 4.

For this workout, we have 6 sets with 60 seconds of rest between each set.

Remember to focus on proper form throughout your sets.

Sets:

1. 18 dips
2. 18 dips
3. 18 dips
4. 18 dips
5. 18 dips
6. 2 fundamental dips with a 5 second descend.

If you completed this workout, head to Greenhorn Group Workout 5 for your next session. If not, stick with this one until you complete it.

Glasses of water drank today: 1-2-3-4-5-6-7-8-9-10

Hours of sleep last night: 1-2-3-4-5-6-7-8-9-10

Diet: junk food—————semi-healthy—————healthy

Greenhorn Group Workout 5

Welcome to the Greenhorn Group Workout 5.

For this workout, we have 6 sets with 60 seconds of rest between each set.

Remember to focus on proper form throughout your sets.

Sets:

1. 21 dips
2. 21 dips
3. 21 dips
4. 21 dips
5. 21 dips
6. 2 fundamental dips with a 5 second descend.

If you completed this workout, head to Greenhorn Group Workout 6 for your next session. If not, stick with this one until you complete it.

Glasses of water drank today: 1-2-3-4-5-6-7-8-9-10

Hours of sleep last night: 1-2-3-4-5-6-7-8-9-10

Diet: junk food————semi-healthy————healthy

Greenhorn Group Workout 6

Welcome to the Greenhorn Group Workout 6.

For this workout, we have 6 sets with 90 seconds of rest between each set.

Remember to focus on proper form throughout your sets.

Sets:

1. 23 dips
2. 23 dips
3. 23 dips
4. 23 dips
5. 23 dips
6. Max out: perform as many dips as you can.

Max reps: _____

Since this is the end of a two-week period, it is time to redo your dip assessment to check your progress if you fully completed this workout.

Rest a day and give the assessment a go to see which Group you will be in next.

Glasses of water drank today: 1-2-3-4-5-6-7-8-9-10

Hours of sleep last night: 1-2-3-4-5-6-7-8-9-10

Diet: junk food———––semi-healthy———––healthy

Cub Group Workouts

Cub Group Workout 1

Welcome to the Cub Group Workout 1.

For this workout, we have 6 sets with 60 seconds of rest between each set.

Remember to focus on proper form throughout your sets.

Sets:

1. 17 dips
2. 17 dips
3. 17 dips
4. 17 dips
5. 17 dips
6. 1 fundamental dip with a 10 second descend.

If you completed this workout, head to Cub Group Workout 2 for your next session. If not, stick with this one until you complete it.

Glasses of water drank today: 1-2-3-4-5-6-7-8-9-10

Hours of sleep last night: 1-2-3-4-5-6-7-8-9-10

Diet: junk food—————semi-healthy—————healthy

Cub Group Workout 2

Welcome to the Cub Group Workout 2.

For this workout, we have 6 sets with 60 seconds of rest between each set.

Remember to focus on proper form throughout your sets.

Sets:

1. 18 dips
2. 18 dips
3. 18 dips
4. 18 dips
5. 18 dips
6. 1 fundamental dip with a 10 second descend.

If you completed this workout, head to Cub Group Workout 3 for your next session. If not, stick with this one until you complete it.

Glasses of water drank today: 1-2-3-4-5-6-7-8-9-10

Hours of sleep last night: 1-2-3-4-5-6-7-8-9-10

Diet: junk food————semi-healthy————healthy

Cub Group Workout 3

Welcome to the Cub Group Workout 3.

For this workout, we have 6 sets with 90 seconds of rest between each set.

Remember to focus on proper form throughout your sets.

Sets:

1. 21 dips
2. 21 dips
3. 21 dips
4. 21 dips
5. 21 dips
6. Max out: perform as many dips as you can.

Max reps: _____

If you completed this workout, head to Cub Group Workout 4 for your next session. If not, stick with this one until you complete it.

Glasses of water drank today: 1-2-3-4-5-6-7-8-9-10

Hours of sleep last night: 1-2-3-4-5-6-7-8-9-10

Diet: junk food— — — — —semi-healthy— — — — —healthy

Cub Group Workout 4

Welcome to the Cub Group Workout 4.

For this workout, we have 6 sets with 60 seconds of rest between each set.

Remember to focus on proper form throughout your sets.

Sets:

1. 23 dips
2. 23 dips
3. 23 dips
4. 23 dips
5. 23 dips
6. 1 fundamental dip with a 10 second descend.

If you completed this workout, head to Cub Group Workout 5 for your next session. If not, stick with this one until you complete it.

Glasses of water drank today: 1-2-3-4-5-6-7-8-9-10

Hours of sleep last night: 1-2-3-4-5-6-7-8-9-10

Diet: junk food———————semi-healthy———————healthy

Cub Group Workout 5

Welcome to the Cub Group Workout 5.

For this workout, we have 6 sets with 60 seconds of rest between each set.

Remember to focus on proper form throughout your sets.

Sets:

1. 26 dips
2. 26 dips
3. 26 dips
4. 26 dips
5. 26 dips
6. 1 fundamental dip with a 10 second descend.

If you completed this workout, head to Cub Group Workout 6 for your next session. If not, stick with this one until you complete it.

Glasses of water drank today: 1-2-3-4-5-6-7-8-9-10

Hours of sleep last night: 1-2-3-4-5-6-7-8-9-10

Diet: junk food—————semi-healthy—————healthy

Cub Group Workout 6

Welcome to the Cub Group Workout 6.

For this workout, we have 6 sets with 90 seconds of rest between each set.

Remember to focus on proper form throughout your sets.

Sets:

1. 27 dips
2. 27 dips
3. 27 dips
4. 27 dips
5. 27 dips
6. Max out: perform as many dips as you can.

Max reps: _____

Since this is the end of a two-week period, it is time to redo your dip assessment to check your progress if you fully completed this workout.

Rest a day and give the assessment a go to see which Group you will be in next.

Glasses of water drank today: 1-2-3-4-5-6-7-8-9-10

Hours of sleep last night: 1-2-3-4-5-6-7-8-9-10

Diet: junk food————semi-healthy————healthy

Rookie Group Workouts

Rookie Group Workout 1

Welcome to the Rookie Group Workout 1.

For this workout, we have 6 sets with 60 seconds of rest between each set.

Remember to focus on proper form throughout your sets.

Sets:

1. 21 dips
2. 21 dips
3. 21 dips
4. 21 dips
5. 21 dips
6. 1 fundamental dip with a 10 second descend.

If you completed this workout, head to Cub Group Workout 2 for your next session. If not, stick with this one until you complete it.

Glasses of water drank today: 1-2-3-4-5-6-7-8-9-10

Hours of sleep last night: 1-2-3-4-5-6-7-8-9-10

Diet: junk food————semi-healthy————healthy

Rookie Group Workout 2

Welcome to the Rookie Group Workout 2.

For this workout, we have 6 sets with 60 seconds of rest between each set.

Remember to focus on proper form throughout your sets.

Sets:

1. 23 dips
2. 23 dips
3. 23 dips
4. 23 dips
5. 23 dips
6. 1 fundamental dip with a 10 second descend.

If you completed this workout, head to Rookie Group Workout 3 for your next session. If not, stick with this one until you complete it.

Glasses of water drank today: 1-2-3-4-5-6-7-8-9-10

Hours of sleep last night: 1-2-3-4-5-6-7-8-9-10

Diet: junk food—————semi-healthy—————healthy

Rookie Group Workout 3

Welcome to the Rookie Group Workout 3.

For this workout, we have 6 sets with 90 seconds of rest between each set.

Remember to focus on proper form throughout your sets.

Sets:

1. 26 dips
2. 26 dips
3. 26 dips
4. 26 dips
5. 26 dips
6. Max out: perform as many dips as you can.

Max reps: _____

If you completed this workout, head to Rookie Group Workout 4 for your next session. If not, stick with this one until you complete it.

Glasses of water drank today: 1-2-3-4-5-6-7-8-9-10

Hours of sleep last night: 1-2-3-4-5-6-7-8-9-10

Diet: junk food—————semi-healthy—————healthy

Rookie Group Workout 4

Welcome to the Rookie Group Workout 4.

For this workout, we have 6 sets with 60 seconds of rest between each set.

Remember to focus on proper form throughout your sets.

Sets:

1. 27 dips
2. 27 dips
3. 27 dips
4. 27 dips
5. 27 dips
6. 2 fundamental dips with a 10 second descend.

If you completed this workout, head to Rookie Group Workout 5 for your next session. If not, stick with this one until you complete it.

Glasses of water drank today: 1-2-3-4-5-6-7-8-9-10

Hours of sleep last night: 1-2-3-4-5-6-7-8-9-10

Diet: junk food—————semi-healthy—————healthy

Rookie Group Workout 5

Welcome to the Rookie Group Workout 5.

For this workout, we have 6 sets with 60 seconds of rest between each set.

Remember to focus on proper form throughout your sets.

Sets:

1. 33 dips
2. 33 dips
3. 33 dips
4. 33 dips
5. 33 dips
6. 2 fundamental dips with a 10 second descend.

If you completed this workout, head to Rookie Group Workout 6 for your next session. If not, stick with this one until you complete it.

Glasses of water drank today: 1-2-3-4-5-6-7-8-9-10

Hours of sleep last night: 1-2-3-4-5-6-7-8-9-10

Diet: junk food————semi-healthy————healthy

Rookie Group Workout 6

Welcome to the Rookie Group Workout 6.

For this workout, we have 6 sets with 90 seconds of rest between each set.

Remember to focus on proper form throughout your sets.

Sets:

1. 37 dips
2. 37 dips
3. 37 dips
4. 37 dips
5. 37 dips
6. Max out: perform as many dips as you can.

Max reps: _____

Since this is the end of a two-week period, it is time to redo your dip assessment to check your progress if you fully completed this workout.

Rest a day and give the assessment a go to see which Group you will be in next.

Glasses of water drank today: 1-2-3-4-5-6-7-8-9-10

Hours of sleep last night: 1-2-3-4-5-6-7-8-9-10

Diet: junk food———––semi-healthy———––healthy

Pleb Group Workouts

Pleb Group Workout 1

Welcome to the Pleb Group Workout 1.

For this workout, we have 6 sets with 60 seconds of rest between each set.

Remember to focus on proper form throughout your sets.

Sets:

1. 26 dips
2. 26 dips
3. 26 dips
4. 26 dips
5. 26 dips
6. 1 fundamental dip1 with a 10 second descend.

If you completed this workout, head to Pleb Group Workout 2 for your next session. If not, stick with this one until you complete it.

Glasses of water drank today: 1-2-3-4-5-6-7-8-9-10

Hours of sleep last night: 1-2-3-4-5-6-7-8-9-10

Diet: junk food—————semi-healthy—————healthy

Pleb Group Workout 2

Welcome to the Pleb Group Workout 2.

For this workout, we have 6 sets with 60 seconds of rest between each set.

Remember to focus on proper form throughout your sets.

Sets:

1. 29 dips
2. 29 dips
3. 29 dips
4. 29 dips
5. 29 dips
6. 2 fundamental dips with a 10 second descend.

If you completed this workout, head to Pleb Group Workout 3 for your next session. If not, stick with this one until you complete it.

Glasses of water drank today: 1-2-3-4-5-6-7-8-9-10

Hours of sleep last night: 1-2-3-4-5-6-7-8-9-10

Diet: junk food—————semi-healthy—————healthy

Pleb Group Workout 3

Welcome to the Pleb Group Workout 3.

For this workout, we have 6 sets with 90 seconds of rest between each set.

Remember to focus on proper form throughout your sets.

Sets:

1. 32 dips
2. 32 dips
3. 32 dips
4. 32 dips
5. 32 dips
6. Max out: perform as many dips as you can.

Max reps: _____

If you completed this workout, head to Pleb Group Workout 4 for your next session. If not, stick with this one until you complete it.

Glasses of water drank today: 1-2-3-4-5-6-7-8-9-10

Hours of sleep last night: 1-2-3-4-5-6-7-8-9-10

Diet: junk food—————semi-healthy—————healthy

Pleb Group Workout 4

Welcome to the Pleb Group Workout 4.

For this workout, we have 6 sets with 60 seconds of rest between each set.

Remember to focus on proper form throughout your sets.

Sets:

1. 33 dips
2. 33 dips
3. 33 dips
4. 33 dips
5. 33 dips
6. 2 fundamental dips with a 10 second descend.

If you completed this workout, head to Pleb Group Workout 5 for your next session. If not, stick with this one until you complete it.

Glasses of water drank today: 1-2-3-4-5-6-7-8-9-10

Hours of sleep last night: 1-2-3-4-5-6-7-8-9-10

Diet: junk food————semi-healthy————healthy

Pleb Group Workout 5

Welcome to the Pleb Group Workout 5.

For this workout, we have 6 sets with 60 seconds of rest between each set.

Remember to focus on proper form throughout your sets.

Sets:

1. 39 dips
2. 39 dips
3. 39 dips
4. 39 dips
5. 39 dips
6. 2 fundamental dips with a 10 second descend.

If you completed this workout, head to Pleb Group Workout 6 for your next session. If not, stick with this one until you complete it.

Glasses of water drank today: 1-2-3-4-5-6-7-8-9-10

Hours of sleep last night: 1-2-3-4-5-6-7-8-9-10

Diet: junk food————semi-healthy————healthy

Pleb Group Workout 6

Welcome to the Pleb Group Workout 6.

For this workout, we have 6 sets with 90 seconds of rest between each set.

Remember to focus on proper form throughout your sets.

Sets:

1. 45 dips
2. 45 dips
3. 45 dips
4. 45 dips
5. 45 dips
6. Max out: perform as many dips as you can.

Max reps: _____

Since this is the end of a two-week period, it is time to redo your dip assessment to check your progress if you fully completed this workout.

Rest a day and give the assessment a go to see which Group you will be in next.

Glasses of water drank today: 1-2-3-4-5-6-7-8-9-10

Hours of sleep last night: 1-2-3-4-5-6-7-8-9-10

Diet: junk food—————semi-healthy—————healthy

Gorilla Group Workouts

Gorilla Group Workout 1

Welcome to the Gorilla Group Workout 1.

For this workout, we have 6 sets with 120 seconds of rest between each set.

Remember to focus on proper form throughout your sets.

Sets:

1. 32 dips
2. 32 dips
3. 32 dips
4. 32 dips
5. 32 dips
6. 1 fundamental dip with a 10 second descend.

If you completed this workout, head to Gorilla Group Workout 2 for your next session. If not, stick with this one until you complete it.

Glasses of water drank today: 1-2-3-4-5-6-7-8-9-10

Hours of sleep last night: 1-2-3-4-5-6-7-8-9-10

Diet: junk food————semi-healthy————healthy

Gorilla Group Workout 2

Welcome to the Gorilla Group Workout 2.

For this workout, we have 9 sets with 90 seconds of rest between each set.

Remember to focus on proper form throughout your sets.

Sets:

1. 20 dips
2. 20 dips
3. 20 dips
4. 20 dips
5. 20 dips
6. 20 dips
7. 20 dips
8. 20 dips
9. 2 fundamental dips with a 10 second descend.

If you completed this workout, head to Gorilla Group Workout 3 for your next session. If not, stick with this one until you complete it.

Glasses of water drank today: 1-2-3-4-5-6-7-8-9-10

Hours of sleep last night: 1-2-3-4-5-6-7-8-9-10

Diet: junk food————semi-healthy————healthy

Gorilla Group Workout 3

Welcome to the Gorilla Group Workout 3.

For this workout, we have 9 sets with 90 seconds of rest between each set.

Remember to focus on proper form throughout your sets.

Sets:

1. 23 dips
2. 23 dips
3. 23 dips
4. 23 dips
5. 23 dips
6. 23 dips
7. 23 dips
8. 23 dips
9. Max out: perform as many dips as you can.

Max reps: _____

If you completed this workout, head to Gorilla Group Workout 4 for your next session. If not, stick with this one until you complete it.

Glasses of water drank today: 1-2-3-4-5-6-7-8-9-10

Hours of sleep last night: 1-2-3-4-5-6-7-8-9-10

Diet: junk food————semi-healthy————healthy

Gorilla Group Workout 4

Welcome to the Gorilla Group Workout 4.

For this workout, we have 6 sets with 120 seconds of rest between each set.

Remember to focus on proper form throughout your sets.

Sets:

1. 45 dips
2. 45 dips
3. 45 dips
4. 45 dips
5. 45 dips
6. 3 fundamental dips with a 10 second descend.

If you completed this workout, head to Gorilla Group Workout 5 for your next session. If not, stick with this one until you complete it.

Glasses of water drank today: 1-2-3-4-5-6-7-8-9-10

Hours of sleep last night: 1-2-3-4-5-6-7-8-9-10

Diet: junk food—————semi-healthy—————healthy

Gorilla Group Workout 5

Welcome to the Gorilla Group Workout 5.

For this workout, we have 10 sets with 90 seconds of rest between each set.

Remember to focus on proper form throughout your sets.

Sets:

1. 26 dips
2. 26 dips
3. 26 dips
4. 26 dips
5. 26 dips
6. 26 dips
7. 26 dips
8. 26 dips
9. 26 dips
10. 3 fundamental dips with a 10 second descend.

If you completed this workout, head to Gorilla Group Workout 6 for your next session. If not, stick with this one until you complete it.

Glasses of water drank today: 1-2-3-4-5-6-7-8-9-10

Hours of sleep last night: 1-2-3-4-5-6-7-8-9-10

Diet: junk food————semi-healthy————healthy

Gorilla Group Workout 6

Welcome to the Gorilla Group Workout 6.

For this workout, we have 10 sets with 90 seconds of rest between each set.

Remember to focus on proper form throughout your sets.

Sets:

1. 28 dips
2. 28 dips
3. 28 dips
4. 28 dips
5. 28 dips
6. 28 dips
7. 28 dips
8. 28 dips
9. 28 dips
10. Max out: perform as many dips as you can.

Max reps: _____

Since this is the end of a two-week period, it is time to redo your dip assessment to check your progress if you fully completed this workout.

Rest a day and give the assessment a go to see which Group you will be in next.

Glasses of water drank today: 1-2-3-4-5-6-7-8-9-10

Hours of sleep last night: 1-2-3-4-5-6-7-8-9-10

Diet: junk food————semi-healthy————healthy

Viking Group Workouts

Viking Group Workout 1

Welcome to the Viking Group Workout 1.

For this workout, we have 6 sets with 120 seconds of rest between each set.

Remember to focus on proper form throughout your sets.

Sets:

1. 42 dips
2. 42 dips
3. 42 dips
4. 42 dips
5. 42 dips
6. 2 fundamental dips with a 10 second descend.

If you completed this workout, head to Viking Group Workout 2 for your next session. If not, stick with this one until you complete it.

Glasses of water drank today: 1-2-3-4-5-6-7-8-9-10

Hours of sleep last night: 1-2-3-4-5-6-7-8-9-10

Diet: junk food—————semi-healthy—————healthy

Viking Group Workout 2

Welcome to the Viking Group Workout 2.

For this workout, we have 9 sets with 90 seconds of rest between each set.

Remember to focus on proper form throughout your sets.

Sets:

1. 26 dips
2. 26 dips
3. 26 dips
4. 26 dips
5. 26 dips
6. 26 dips
7. 26 dips
8. 26 dips
9. 3 fundamental dips with a 10 second descend.

If you completed this workout, head to Viking Group Workout 3 for your next session. If not, stick with this one until you complete it.

Glasses of water drank today: 1-2-3-4-5-6-7-8-9-10

Hours of sleep last night: 1-2-3-4-5-6-7-8-9-10

Diet: junk food————semi-healthy————healthy

Viking Group Workout 3

Welcome to the Viking Group Workout 3.

For this workout, we have 9 sets with 90 seconds of rest between each set.

Remember to focus on proper form throughout your sets.

Sets:

1. 28 dips
2. 28 dips
3. 28 dips
4. 28 dips
5. 28 dips
6. 28 dips
7. 28 dips
8. 28 dips
9. Max out: perform as many dips as you can.

Max reps: _____

If you completed this workout, head to Viking Group Workout 4 for your next session. If not, stick with this one until you complete it.

Glasses of water drank today: 1-2-3-4-5-6-7-8-9-10

Hours of sleep last night: 1-2-3-4-5-6-7-8-9-10

Diet: junk food—————semi-healthy—————healthy

Viking Group Workout 4

Welcome to the Viking Group Workout 4.

For this workout, we have 6 sets with 120 seconds of rest between each set.

Remember to focus on proper form throughout your sets.

Sets:

1. 53 dips
2. 53 dips
3. 53 dips
4. 53 dips
5. 53 dips
6. 3 fundamental dips with a 10 second descend.

If you completed this workout, head to Viking Group Workout 5 for your next session. If not, stick with this one until you complete it.

Glasses of water drank today: 1-2-3-4-5-6-7-8-9-10

Hours of sleep last night: 1-2-3-4-5-6-7-8-9-10

Diet: junk food————semi-healthy————healthy

Viking Group Workout 5

Welcome to the Viking Group Workout 5.

For this workout, we have 10 sets with 90 seconds of rest between each set.

Remember to focus on proper form throughout your sets.

Sets:

1. 31 dips
2. 31 dips
3. 31 dips
4. 31 dips
5. 31 dips
6. 31 dips
7. 31 dips
8. 31 dips
9. 31 dips
10. 4 fundamental dips with a 10 second descend.

If you completed this workout, head to Viking Group Workout 6 for your next session. If not, stick with this one until you complete it.

Glasses of water drank today: 1-2-3-4-5-6-7-8-9-10

Hours of sleep last night: 1-2-3-4-5-6-7-8-9-10

Diet: junk food—————semi-healthy—————healthy

Viking Group Workout 6

Welcome to the Viking Group Workout 6.

For this workout, we have 10 sets with 90 seconds of rest between each set.

Remember to focus on proper form throughout your sets.

Sets:

1. 36 dips
2. 36 dips
3. 36 dips
4. 36 dips
5. 36 dips
6. 36 dips
7. 36 dips
8. 36 dips
9. 36 dips
10. Max out: perform as many dips as you can.

Max reps: _____

Since this is the end of a two-week period, it is time to redo your dips assessment to check your progress if you fully completed this workout.

Rest a day and give the assessment a go to see which Group you will be in next.

Glasses of water drank today: 1-2-3-4-5-6-7-8-9-10

Hours of sleep last night: 1-2-3-4-5-6-7-8-9-10

Diet: junk food————semi-healthy————healthy

Elite Group Workouts

Elite Group Workout 1

Welcome to the Elite Group Workout 1.

For this workout, we have 6 sets with 120 seconds of rest between each set.

Remember to focus on proper form throughout your sets.

Sets:

1. 49 dips
2. 49 dips
3. 49 dips
4. 49 dips
5. 49 dips
6. 3 fundamental dips with a 10 second descend.

If you completed this workout, head to Elite Group Workout 2 for your next session. If not, stick with this one until you complete it.

Glasses of water drank today: 1-2-3-4-5-6-7-8-9-10

Hours of sleep last night: 1-2-3-4-5-6-7-8-9-10

Diet: junk food————semi-healthy————healthy

Elite Group Workout 2

Welcome to the Elite Group Workout 2.

For this workout, we have 9 sets with 90 seconds of rest between each set.

Remember to focus on proper form throughout your sets.

Sets:

1. 30 dips
2. 30 dips
3. 30 dips
4. 30 dips
5. 30 dips
6. 30 dips
7. 30 dips
8. 30 dips
9. 3 fundamental dips with a 10 second descend.

If you completed this workout, head to Elite Group Workout 3 for your next session. If not, stick with this one until you complete it.

Glasses of water drank today: 1-2-3-4-5-6-7-8-9-10

Hours of sleep last night: 1-2-3-4-5-6-7-8-9-10

Diet: junk food————semi-healthy————healthy

Elite Group Workout 3

Welcome to the Elite Group Workout 3.

For this workout, we have 9 sets with 90 seconds of rest between each set.

Remember to focus on proper form throughout your sets.

Sets:

1. 33 dips
2. 33 dips
3. 33 dips
4. 33 dips
5. 33 dips
6. 33 dips
7. 33 dips
8. 33 dips
9. Max out: perform as many dips as you can.

Max reps: _____

If you completed this workout, head to Elite Group Workout 4 for your next session. If not, stick with this one until you complete it.

Glasses of water drank today: 1-2-3-4-5-6-7-8-9-10

Hours of sleep last night: 1-2-3-4-5-6-7-8-9-10

Diet: junk food—————semi-healthy—————healthy

Elite Group Workout 4

Welcome to the Elite Group Workout 4.

For this workout, we have 6 sets with 120 seconds of rest between each set.

Remember to focus on proper form throughout your sets.

Sets:

1. 62 dips
2. 62 dips
3. 62 dips
4. 62 dips
5. 62 dips
6. 4 fundamental dips with a 10 second descend.

If you completed this workout, head to Elite Group Workout 5 for your next session. If not, stick with this one until you complete it.

Glasses of water drank today: 1-2-3-4-5-6-7-8-9-10

Hours of sleep last night: 1-2-3-4-5-6-7-8-9-10

Diet: junk food————semi-healthy————healthy

Elite Group Workout 5

Welcome to the Elite Group Workout 5.

For this workout, we have 10 sets with 90 seconds of rest between each set.

Remember to focus on proper form throughout your sets.

Sets:

1. 36 dips
2. 36 dips
3. 36 dips
4. 36 dips
5. 36 dips
6. 36 dips
7. 36 dips
8. 36 dips
9. 36 dips
10. 4 fundamental dips with a 10 second descend.

If you completed this workout, head to Elite Group Workout 6 for your next session. If not, stick with this one until you complete it.

Glasses of water drank today: 1-2-3-4-5-6-7-8-9-10

Hours of sleep last night: 1-2-3-4-5-6-7-8-9-10

Diet: junk food———— semi-healthy———— healthy

Elite Group Workout 6

Welcome to the Elite Group Workout 6.

For this workout, we have 10 sets with 90 seconds of rest between each set.

Remember to focus on proper form throughout your sets.

Sets:

1. 41 dips
2. 41 dips
3. 41 dips
4. 41 dips
5. 41 dips
6. 41 dips
7. 41 dips
8. 41 dips
9. 41 dips
10. Max out: perform as many dips as you can.

Max reps: _____

Since this is the end of a two-week period, it is time to redo your dip assessment to check your progress if you fully completed this workout.

Rest a day and give the assessment a go to see which Group you will be in next.

Glasses of water drank today: 1-2-3-4-5-6-7-8-9-10

Hours of sleep last night: 1-2-3-4-5-6-7-8-9-10

Diet: junk food————semi-healthy————healthy

Commando Group Workouts

Commando Group Workout 1

Welcome to the Commando Group Workout 1.

For this workout, we have 6 sets with 120 seconds of rest between each set.

Remember to focus on proper form throughout your sets.

Sets:

1. 53 dips
2. 53 dips
3. 53 dips
4. 53 dips
5. 53 dips
6. 4 fundamental dips with a 10 second descend.

If you completed this workout, head to Commando Group Workout 2 for your next session. If not, stick with this one until you complete it.

Glasses of water drank today: 1-2-3-4-5-6-7-8-9-10

Hours of sleep last night: 1-2-3-4-5-6-7-8-9-10

Diet: junk food————semi-healthy————healthy

Commando Group Workout 2

Welcome to the Commando Group Workout 2.

For this workout, we have 10 sets with 90 seconds of rest between each set.

Remember to focus on proper form throughout your sets.

Sets:

1. 31 dips
2. 31 dips
3. 31 dips
4. 31 dips
5. 31 dips
6. 31 dips
7. 31 dips
8. 31 dips
9. 31 dips
10. 4 fundamental dips with a 10 second descend.

If you completed this workout, head to Commando Group Workout 3 for your next session. If not, stick with this one until you complete it.

Glasses of water drank today: 1-2-3-4-5-6-7-8-9-10

Hours of sleep last night: 1-2-3-4-5-6-7-8-9-10

Diet: junk food————semi-healthy————healthy

Commando Group Workout 3

Welcome to the Commando Group Workout 3.

For this workout, we have 10 sets with 90 seconds of rest between each set.

Remember to focus on proper form throughout your sets.

Sets:

1. 34 dips
2. 34 dips
3. 34 dips
4. 34 dips
5. 34 dips
6. 34 dips
7. 34 dips
8. 34 dips
9. 34 dips
10. Max out: perform as many dips as you can.

Max reps: _____

If you completed this workout, head to Commando Group Workout 4 for your next session. If not, stick with this one until you complete it.

Glasses of water drank today: 1-2-3-4-5-6-7-8-9-10

Hours of sleep last night: 1-2-3-4-5-6-7-8-9-10

Diet: junk food————semi-healthy————healthy

Commando Group Workout 4

Welcome to the Commando Group Workout 4.

For this workout, we have 6 sets with 120 seconds of rest between each set.

Remember to focus on proper form throughout your sets.

Sets:

1. 74 dips
2. 74 dips
3. 74 dips
4. 74 dips
5. 74 dips
6. 5 fundamental dips with a 10 second descend.

If you completed this workout, head to Commando Group Workout 5 for your next session. If not, stick with this one until you complete it.

Glasses of water drank today: 1-2-3-4-5-6-7-8-9-10

Hours of sleep last night: 1-2-3-4-5-6-7-8-9-10

Diet: junk food————semi-healthy————healthy

Commando Group Workout 5

Welcome to the Commando Group Workout 5.

For this workout, we have 10 sets with 90 seconds of rest between each set.

Remember to focus on proper form throughout your sets.

Sets:

1. 36 dips
2. 36 dips
3. 36 dips
4. 36 dips
5. 36 dips
6. 36 dips
7. 36 dips
8. 36 dips
9. 36 dips
10. 5 fundamental dips with a 10 second descend.

If you completed this workout, head to Commando Group Workout 6 for your next session. If not, stick with this one until you complete it.

Glasses of water drank today: 1-2-3-4-5-6-7-8-9-10

Hours of sleep last night: 1-2-3-4-5-6-7-8-9-10

Diet: junk food————semi-healthy————healthy

Commando Group Workout 6

Welcome to the Commando Group Workout 6.

For this workout, we have 10 sets with 90 seconds of rest between each set.

Remember to focus on proper form throughout your sets.

Sets:

1. 42 dips
2. 42 dips
3. 42 dips
4. 42 dips
5. 42 dips
6. 42 dips
7. 42 dips
8. 42 dips
9. 42 dips
10. Max out: perform as many dips as you can.

Max reps: _____

If you completed this workout, you have earned the right to attempt hitting 150 consecutive dips. Take a few days off to fully recover and take a shot at

hitting your goal.

You got this.

Glasses of water drank today: 1-2-3-4-5-6-7-8-9-10

Hours of sleep last night: 1-2-3-4-5-6-7-8-9-10

Diet: junk food————semi-healthy————healthy

Veteran Group Workouts

Veteran Group Workout 1

Welcome to the Veteran Group Workout 1.

For this workout, we have 6 sets with 120 seconds of rest between each set.

Remember to focus on proper form throughout your sets.

Sets:

1. 65 dips
2. 65 dips
3. 65 dips
4. 65 dips
5. 65 dips
6. 4 fundamental dips with a 10 second descend.

If you completed this workout, head to Veteran Group Workout 2 for your next session. If not, stick with this one until you complete it.

Glasses of water drank today: 1-2-3-4-5-6-7-8-9-10

Hours of sleep last night: 1-2-3-4-5-6-7-8-9-10

Diet: junk food————semi-healthy————healthy

Veteran Group Workout 2

Welcome to the Veteran Group Workout 2.

For this workout, we have 10 sets with 90 seconds of rest between each set.

Remember to focus on proper form throughout your sets.

Sets:

1. 34 dips
2. 34 dips
3. 34 dips
4. 34 dips
5. 34 dips
6. 34 dips
7. 34 dips
8. 34 dips
9. 34 dips
10. 4 fundamental dips with a 10 second descend.

If you completed this workout, head to Veteran Group Workout 3 for your next session. If not, stick with this one until you complete it.

Glasses of water drank today: 1-2-3-4-5-6-7-8-9-10

Hours of sleep last night: 1-2-3-4-5-6-7-8-9-10

Diet: junk food————semi-healthy————healthy

Veteran Group Workout 3

Welcome to the Veteran Group Workout 3.

For this workout, we have 10 sets with 90 seconds of rest between each set.

Remember to focus on proper form throughout your sets.

Sets:

1. 39 dips
2. 39 dips
3. 39 dips
4. 39 dips
5. 39 dips
6. 39 dips
7. 39 dips
8. 39 dips
9. 39 dips
10. Max out: perform as many dips as you can.

Max reps: _____

If you completed this workout, head to Veteran Group Workout 4 for your next session. If not, stick with this one until you complete it.

Glasses of water drank today: 1-2-3-4-5-6-7-8-9-10

Hours of sleep last night: 1-2-3-4-5-6-7-8-9-10

Diet: junk food————semi-healthy————healthy

Veteran Group Workout 4

Welcome to the Veteran Group Workout 4.

For this workout, we have 6 sets with 120 seconds of rest between each set.

Remember to focus on proper form throughout your sets.

Sets:

1. 80 dips
2. 80 dips
3. 80 dips
4. 80 dips
5. 80 dips
6. 5 fundamental dips with a 10 second descend.

If you completed this workout, head to Veteran Group Workout 5 for your next session. If not, stick with this one until you complete it.

Glasses of water drank today: 1-2-3-4-5-6-7-8-9-10

Hours of sleep last night: 1-2-3-4-5-6-7-8-9-10

Diet: junk food————semi-healthy————healthy

Veteran Group Workout 5

Welcome to the Veteran Group Workout 5.

For this workout, we have 10 sets with 90 seconds of rest between each set.

Remember to focus on proper form throughout your sets.

Sets:

1. 42 dips
2. 42 dips
3. 42 dips
4. 42 dips
5. 42 dips
6. 42 dips
7. 42 dips
8. 42 dips
9. 42 dips
10. 5 fundamental dips with a 10 second descend.

If you completed this workout, head to Veteran Group Workout 6 for your next session. If not, stick with this one until you complete it.

Glasses of water drank today: 1-2-3-4-5-6-7-8-9-10

Hours of sleep last night: 1-2-3-4-5-6-7-8-9-10

Diet: junk food———————semi-healthy—————healthy

Veteran Group Workout 6

Welcome to the Veteran Group Workout 6.

For this workout, we have 10 sets with 90 seconds of rest between each set.

Remember to focus on proper form throughout your sets.

Sets:

1. 44 dips
2. 44 dips
3. 44 dips
4. 44 dips
5. 44 dips
6. 44 dips
7. 44 dips
8. 44 dips
9. 44 dips
10. Max out: perform as many dips as you can.

Max reps: _____

If you completed this workout, you have earned the right to attempt hitting 150 consecutive dips. Take a few days off to fully recover and take a shot at

hitting your goal.

You got this.

Glasses of water drank today: 1-2-3-4-5-6-7-8-9-10

Hours of sleep last night: 1-2-3-4-5-6-7-8-9-10

Diet: junk food————semi-healthy————healthy

Nuclear Group Workouts

Nuclear Group Workout 1

Welcome to the Nuclear Group Workout 1.

For this workout, we have 6 sets with 120 seconds of rest between each set.

Remember to focus on proper form throughout your sets.

Sets:

1. 74 dips
2. 74 dips
3. 74 dips
4. 74 dips
5. 74 dips
6. 5 fundamental dips with a 10 second descend.

If you completed this workout, head to Nuclear Group Workout 2 for your next session. If not, stick with this one until you complete it.

Glasses of water drank today: 1-2-3-4-5-6-7-8-9-10

Hours of sleep last night: 1-2-3-4-5-6-7-8-9-10

Diet: junk food————semi-healthy————healthy

Nuclear Group Workout 2

Welcome to the Nuclear Group Workout 2.

For this workout, we have 10 sets with 90 seconds of rest between each set.

Remember to focus on proper form throughout your sets.

Sets:

1. 39 dips
2. 39 dips
3. 39 dips
4. 39 dips
5. 39 dips
6. 39 dips
7. 39 dips
8. 39 dips
9. 39 dips
10. 5 fundamental dips with a 10 second descend.

If you completed this workout, head to Nuclear Group Workout 3 for your next session. If not, stick with this one until you complete it.

Glasses of water drank today: 1-2-3-4-5-6-7-8-9-10

Hours of sleep last night: 1-2-3-4-5-6-7-8-9-10

Diet: junk food————semi-healthy————healthy

Nuclear Group Workout 3

Welcome to the Nuclear Group Workout 3.

For this workout, we have 10 sets with 90 seconds of rest between each set.

Remember to focus on proper form throughout your sets.

Sets:

1. 44 dips
2. 44 dips
3. 44 dips
4. 44 dips
5. 44 dips
6. 44 dips
7. 44 dips
8. 44 dips
9. 44 dips
10. Max out: perform as many dips as you can.

Max reps: _____

If you completed this workout, head to Nuclear Group Workout 4 for your next session. If not, stick with this one until you complete it.

Glasses of water drank today: 1-2-3-4-5-6-7-8-9-10

Hours of sleep last night: 1-2-3-4-5-6-7-8-9-10

Diet: junk food————semi-healthy————healthy

Nuclear Group Workout 4

Welcome to the Nuclear Group Workout 4.

For this workout, we have 6 sets with 120 seconds of rest between each set.

Remember to focus on proper form throughout your sets.

Sets:

1. 89 dips
2. 89 dips
3. 89 dips
4. 89 dips
5. 89 dips
6. 5 fundamental dips with a 10 second descend.

If you completed this workout, head to Nuclear Group Workout 5 for your next session. If not, stick with this one until you complete it.

Glasses of water drank today: 1-2-3-4-5-6-7-8-9-10

Hours of sleep last night: 1-2-3-4-5-6-7-8-9-10

Diet: junk food—————semi-healthy—————healthy

Nuclear Group Workout 5

Welcome to the Nuclear Group Workout 5.

For this workout, we have 10 sets with 90 seconds of rest between each set.

Remember to focus on proper form throughout your sets.

Sets:

1. 45 dips
2. 45 dips
3. 45 dips
4. 45 dips
5. 45 dips
6. 45 dips
7. 45 dips
8. 45 dips
9. 45 dips
10. 18 fundamental dips with a 10 second descend.

If you completed this workout, head to Nuclear Group Workout 6 for your next session. If not, stick with this one until you complete it.

Glasses of water drank today: 1-2-3-4-5-6-7-8-9-10

Hours of sleep last night: 1-2-3-4-5-6-7-8-9-10

Diet: junk food—————semi-healthy—————healthy

Nuclear Group Workout 6

Welcome to the Nuclear Group Workout 6.

For this workout, we have 10 sets with 90 seconds of rest between each set.

Remember to focus on proper form throughout your sets.

Sets:

1. 48 dips
2. 48 dips
3. 48 dips
4. 48 dips
5. 48 dips
6. 48 dips
7. 48 dips
8. 48 dips
9. 48 dips
10. Max out: perform as many dips as you can.

Max reps: _____

If you completed this workout, you have earned the right to attempt hitting 150 consecutive dips. Take a few days off to fully recover and take a shot at

hitting your goal.

You got this.

Glasses of water drank today: 1-2-3-4-5-6-7-8-9-10

Hours of sleep last night: 1-2-3-4-5-6-7-8-9-10

Diet: junk food————semi-healthy————healthy

Attempting 150 Consecutive Dips

If you are here, that means you have completed either the Commando, Veteran, or Nuclear Group Workouts and have earned the right to attempt nailing down 150 consecutive dips.

This goal is well within your grasp and all you have to do is take it.

As you begin to warm up to crush this, I would like to ask a favor.

I am going to be greedy for a minute here and ask you to leave a review for the book.

Reviews are a pain to get but it will only take a minute or two to leave one.

Scan this QR code which will take you straight to the book's page on Amazon.

Scroll down and click the 'leave a customer review' button, select your star rating, leave a few words, and that is it!

It is that simple!

Once that is done, get ready to crush this.

Get psyched for what is about to happen.

Now give it everything you got to knock out as many correct dips without stopping.

Once you are done, come back.

* * *

If you nailed 150 or more, awesome.

That is incredible. Time to knock that off your bucket list.

If you did not hit the goal, no worries. Not everyone gets it on the first try.

Use this number as your new assessment number and get back at it!

Cheers.

Conclusion:

I just want to thank you for making your way through this program and the book. You have bettered yourself for it.

I hope you have challenged yourself and I hope you tasted victory by reaching 150 consecutive dips.

If you are hungry for more challenges, we have got plenty more where this came from.

And if you have enjoyed this book, do take a second to leave a review.

Until next time.

Cheers.

Printed in Great Britain
by Amazon

75821168R00090